Contents

Fertility Diet

The fertility diet is designed to help you get pregnant by making several changes to your diet and level of activity. These changes emphasize consuming certain foods believed to boost fertility such as plant protein and full-fat dairy products.

How does The Fertility Diet work?

There's no guarantee you'll get pregnant by following Fertility Diet. However, the diet includes steps that may boost fertility for women with conditions such as ovulation disorders, polycystic ovary syndrome, fibroids or uterine polyps, damaged fallopian tubes, endometriosis and immune system disorders. While male conditions such as low sperm count, sperm defects, twisted spermatic cords and immune disorders can also be factors for infertility, the diet is not designed to address male fertility issues.

How easy is Fertility Diet to follow?

Fertility Diet is fairly easy to follow

Convenience shouldn't be an issue but there might be a learning curve. There are no niche or exotic ingredients to contend with. Still, the dietary changes will take some planning and getting used to, with attention paid to nutritional facts printed on food labels.

Find healthy recipes in this cookbook. The recipes and meal plans in this book do not contain any artificial trans fats. Instead of red meat, the book offers fish, eggs, beans, nuts and whole milk or full-fat dairy products as a source of protein. One example of breakfast includes oatmeal, almonds, blueberries and whole milk, while another consists of whole-wheat toast, almond butter, vanilla soy milk, yogurt, sliced peaches and coffee or tea. Other recommended items include salads packed with beans and peppers; smoothies with whole-milk vanilla yogurt, frozen bananas and honey; vegetables and fruit. Dinners include orange-glazed salmon, grilled Moroccan tuna, chili-spiced shrimp and more fish dishes.

Eating out is manageable. This book suggests eating a low-calorie snack such as dried cranberries, edamame, grapes or string cheese before going to a restaurant. If you're not "starving," you're less likely to gorge on unhealthy choices. Avoid french fries, donuts and other fried foods. Ask the server if the fried foods are cooked with partially hydrogenated oils. If they are, choose roasted vegetables or pecan-crusted dishes instead. After dinner, order a coffee in place of dessert. For special occasions, decide ahead of time how much you should eat, stick with your plan and set practical limits. Another option? Offer to bring a side dish to the party; that way you and your friends can snack healthily.

Save time grocery shopping. Making a list before you go grocery shopping will make meal planning easier. Avoiding the chip and soda aisles will save time.

Feeling full shouldn't be a problem. You should feel full after the diet's prescribed three meals and two snacks a day, which should total approximately 2,000 calories. Slow down when chewing your food to prevent overeating. It takes a few minutes for your body to relay to your brain that it is full.

Get used to different tasting foods. Although you may miss indulging in that juicy steak, your taste buds will thank you for introducing more hearty dishes, such as creamy parsnip-carrot soup, orange-glazed salmon and a vegetarian chili that packs a helping of bell peppers and beans.

How much should you exercise on The Fertility Diet?

Exercise is one of the 10 steps recommended on Fertility Diet. Adding 30 minutes of brisk walking to a modest daily reduction in calories has been proven to help ward off excess weight and improve fertility.

Does The Fertility Diet have any health risks?

No, the Fertility Diet does not pose health risks. Since it mimics other diet and exercise plans geared toward people prone to diabetes and cardiovascular disease, it's a healthful diet for women to consider.

Does The Fertility Diet allow for restrictions and preferences?

Most people can customize the Fertility Diet to fit their needs – just pick a preference for more information.

Vegetarian or Vegan: The Fertility Diet excludes red meat as a source of protein. Therefore, it's fairly simple to tailor this diet for vegetarian dietary choices. However, vegans may find it more difficult to follow with its emphasis on full-fat dairy products each day. Gluten-Free: Gluten-free options are possible. Those with an intolerance can substitute whole-wheat products with other healthful choicesLow-Salt: The diet promotes a low-salt eating pattern and can successfully be tailored to more specific low-salt preferences.

Kosher: All fruits and vegetables are kosher. However, shellfish, included in the Fertility Diet menu plans, is not. Some of these ingredients or recipes can be adjusted to kosher preferences.

Halal: Shrimp, cod, salmon and tuna are all permissible with halal preferences. Any butter made with beef fat is against halal. However, fruit, vegetables, dairy products, grains and cereals, and herbs and spices all jibe with halal guidelines.

What Can You Eat?

• Avoid trans fats. Artificial trans fats have been banned in the United States due to their adverse health effects, but you'll want to try to avoid natural trans fats found in margarine, shortening, and fried foods as well.

• Use more unsaturated vegetable oils, such as olive oil and canola oil.

• Eat more vegetable protein, like beans and nuts, and less animal protein.

• Choose whole grains and other sources of carbohydrates that have "lower, slower effects on blood sugar and insulin" rather than "highly refined carbohydrates that quickly boost blood sugar and insulin."

• Consume milk fat every day in the form of a glass of whole milk, a small dish of ice cream, or a cup of full-fat yogurt, and "temporarily trade in skim milk and low- or no-fat dairy products like cottage cheese and frozen yogurt for their full-fat cousins."

• Take a multivitamin with folic acid—critical to fetal development—and other B vitamins.

• Get plenty of iron from fruits, vegetables, beans, and supplements, but not from red meat.

• Be mindful of what you drink. Avoid sugary sodas and other sugar-laden drinks. Drink coffee, tea, and alcoholic beverages in moderation. Instead, drink water.

• Aim for a healthy weight. If you are overweight, losing between 5% and 10% of your weight can jump-start ovulation, according to the research.

• Start a daily exercise plan, or if you already exercise, work out harder. Still, you shouldn't overdo it, especially if you're potentially underweight, since too much exercise can work against conception.

What to Eat

• Unsaturated vegetable oils, such as olive oil and canola oil

• Vegetable protein from beans and nuts

• Whole grains

• Whole milk, ice cream, or full-fat yogurt

• Iron-rich fruits, vegetables, and beans

What Not to Eat

• Trans fats

• Animal protein, especially red meat

- Highly refined grain products

- Sugar-sweetened beverages

- Coffee and tea (only drink in moderation)

- Alcohol

Sample Shopping List

- Dark leafy greens (spinach, kale, Swiss chard)

- Broccoli, asparagus, zucchini

- Citrus fruits (grapefruit, oranges)

- Berries (raspberries, blueberries, blackberries)

- Bananas, avocados

- Whole-grain bread and pasta

- Brown rice and quinoa

- Tofu, chicken, salmon, canned tuna, sardines, eggs

- Full-fat yogurt, milk, cottage cheese

- Natural ice cream (avoid artificial flavors or high amounts of added sugar)

Sample Meal Plan

Day 1

- Breakfast: 5-Minute Avocado and Egg Toast; 8-ounce glass full-fat milk, 1 banana

- Lunch: 1 cup Vegetarian Southwest Quinoa Salad; 1 apple

- Dinner: Fish Tacos With Spicy Sauce and Sweet and Tangy Grilled Veggie Salsa

Day 2

- Breakfast: 3/4 cup full-fat Greek yogurt topped with fresh berries

- Lunch: Stacked Mediterranean Sandwich; 1 cup Red Curry Lentil Soup with Kale; 5 kalamata olives

- Dinner: Roasted Red Pepper and Spinach Pasta; Roasted Beet and Feta Salad

Day 3

- Breakfast: 1 cup oatmeal topped with walnuts or almonds, shaved coconut, and fruit

- Lunch: 1 cup Tomato Basil Soup; whole-grain crackers; 1/2 cup full-fat cottage cheese

- Dinner: Oven-Baked Salmon With Herbs; roasted asparagus; mixed greens

Pros and Cons

Pros

- Diet is generally healthy

- Plant-based foods are emphasized

- Avoids high-sugar foods

- Steers clear of trans fats

Cons

- Diet requires calorie counting

- Emphasis on full-fat milk products

- May require more meal prep

- Could include too much iron

FERTILTY DIET RECIPES

In this part are recipes to help your fertility

Lentil

Preparation time

40 minutes

INGREDIENTS

- 1 cup dried green, brown, or French lentils

- 2 cups water

- 1 bay leaf, garlic clove, or other seasonings (optional)

- 1/4 to 3/4 teaspoon salt

INSTRUCTIONS

1. Rinse the lentils.

2. Place the lentils in a strainer or colander.

3. Pick over and remove any shriveled lentils, debris, or rocks.

4. Thoroughly rinse under running water.

5. Combine the lentils and water.

6. Transfer the rinsed lentils to a small saucepan and add the water.

7. Add any seasonings being used, but do not add the salt yet.

8. Bring to a rapid simmer, then reduce heat.

9. Bring the water to a rapid simmer over medium-high heat.

10. Reduce the heat to maintain a very gentle simmer.

11. You should only see a few small bubbles and some slight movement in the lentils.

12. Simmer the lentils. Simmer uncovered for 20 to 30 minutes.

13. Add more water as needed to make sure the lentils are just barely covered.

14. Salt the lentils.

15. Lentils are cooked as soon as they are tender and no longer crunchy.

16. Older lentils may take longer to cook and shed their outer skins as they cook.

17. Strain the lentils and remove the bay leaf, if used.

18. Return the lentils to the pan and stir in 1/4 teaspoon salt.

19. Taste and add more salt as needed.

20. Season them with olive oil, lemon juice, vinegar, fresh herbs, or eat them on their own.

21. Lentils can also be added to soups, salads, or other recipes.

EQUIPMENT

- Measuring cups

- Strainer or colander

- Small saucepan

RECIPE NOTES

Storage: Cooked lentils can be refrigerated in an airtight container for up to 4 days.

Quinoa jollof

Preparation time

15 minutes

INGREDIENTS

• Quinoa

• Tomatoes

• Red bell pepper

• Onion

• Ginger

- Garlic

- Vegetable broth

- Bouillon cube

- Olive oil

- Tomato paste

- Curry powder

- Thyme

- Cayenne pepper

INSTRUCTIONS

1. Wash quinoa and set aside.

2. Place tomatoes, bell pepper, ½ of onion, ginger, garlic, and vegetable broth in a high-speed blender and process until smooth.

3. Pour liquid mixture and vegan bouillon into a saucepan over medium-high heat, and bring to a boil. Reduce heat to low and simmer for about 10 minutes. Set aside.

4. Heat oil in a large saucepan, add the remaining onion and saute until soft, about 2 minutes.

5. Stir in curry powder, thyme, and cayenne pepper, and cook until fragrant.

6. Add quinoa and stir to coat. Stir in the reduced liquid and add salt to taste.

7. Bring to a boil, then reduce heat to low and simmer for 20 minutes.

Greek yogurt

Preparation time

6 hours 30 minutes

INGREDIENTS

- 4 cups whole milk 960 mL

- ¼ cup plain store bought yogurt ensure the container says "live" or "active" cultures, 60 g

INSTRUCTIONS

1. Heat Milk: Place milk in a medium pot and heat to 185-200°F (85-93°C), stirring frequently to preventing a skin from forming.

2. Cool Bath: Transfer the pot with milk to an ice bath (I filled my sink with ice and water), to cool milk to 100-110°F (37-43°C).

3. Pour ½ cup of the warm milk into a separate clean jar or bowl. Mix in plain yogurt, stirring until yogurt is well blended. Add remaining milk and mix well.

4. Let Sit: Cover jar or bowl with a lid, wrap in a moist, warm towel to keep in heat, and place in oven. Turn on oven light to keep warm, and let

the bacteria do its yogurt making magic for 4 to 8 hours (or overnight).*

5. Strain: You can eat the yogurt like this, or strain it to make Greek yogurt. To strain, line a mesh sieve with cheesecloth (or paper towels, coffee filters etc), and pour yogurt in. Place over a large bowl and let strain in the fridge for a few hours (or overnight), until it's reach a consistency you like.

Pomegranate juice

Preparation time

30 minutes

INGREDIENTS

- 5 to 6 large pomegranates

INSTRUCTIONS

1. Using a paring knife, remove the part of the pomegranate that looks like a crown. I like angling my paring knife downward and making a circle around the crown.

2. Score the pomegranate into sections. I find scoring the fruit 4 times is enough for me, but feel free to score it a few more times.

3. Break open the pomegranate into sections.

4. Fill a large bowl with cool water. Break apart the pomegranate arils underneath the water. It

helps prevent pomegranate juice from squirting everywhere. (By the way, don't wear light colored clothes while you're doing this.) Drain the water from the pomegranate arils when you're done separating them from the rind.

5. Pour the arils into a blender. Blend until all the arils have been crushed but most of the seeds are still in tact. This usually takes no more than 15 to 20 seconds.

6. Pour the juice through a strainer. You'll notice that the juice passes through the strainer pretty slowly because the pulp is pretty thick. To speed up the process, use a rubber spatula to press the pulp agains the strainer. The juice should drip through faster.

7. Pour juice into a glass to serve.

Note

- 5 to 6 large pomegranates should yield about 4 cups of juice. Leftover juice can be refrigerated in a jar for 5 to 6 days.

Bok coy

Preparation time

INGREDIENTS

- 1 pound baby bok choy

- 2 tablespoon soy sauce

- 2 tablespoons vegetable broth

- 1 tablespoon rice vinegar

- 1 tablespoon sesame oil, divided

- 1 teaspoon honey

- ⅛ teaspoon red chili flakes

- 2 tablespoons vegetable oil, divided

- 1 tablespoon minced garlic

- 2 teaspoons minced ginger

- ¼ cup thinly sliced green onions, white and green parts

- ¼ teaspoon sesame seeds

INSTRUCTIONS

1. Rinse the bok choy with water.

2. Shaking off any excess water and then dry using a kitchen towel or paper towels.

3. Cut each bok choy, halved lengthwise.

4. In a small bowl combine soy sauce, broth, vinegar, 2 teaspoons of sesame oil, honey, and red chili flakes.

5. In a wok or 12-inch nonstick skillet add 1 tablespoon vegetable oil and 1 teaspoon of sesame oil over high heat until just smoking.

6. Use tongs to carefully place the bok choy cut side down in a single layer in the wok, lightly press down to make contact with the surface.

7. Cook until lightly browned without moving, about 1 to 2 minutes.

8. Flip the bok choy over and cook the other side until lightly browned, 1 to 2 minutes. Transfer to a plate.

9. Add 1 tablespoon vegetable oil to the wok.

10. Add garlic, ginger and green onions, stir fry until fragrant, about 30 seconds.

11. Add the soy sauce mixture to the wok, simmer until thickened, about 30 seconds.

12. Add bok choy back to the wok, stir-fry and cook until the sauce glazes the greens, about 1 to 2 minutes.

13. Transfer to a platter and garnish with sesame seeds.

Equipment

• Wok

• Wok Spatula

• Colander

Notes

• Make it Gluten-Free: Use coconut aminos, or gluten-free tamari instead of soy sauce.

• Make it Paleo: Use coconut aminos instead of soy sauce, olive oil instead of vegetable oil, and maple syrup instead of honey.

Swiss chard

Preparation time

20 minutes

INGREDIENTS

- 1 large bunch of fresh Swiss chard

- 2 tablespoons extra virgin olive oil

- 1 clove garlic, sliced

- Pinch of dried crushed red pepper

- 1/4 teaspoon of whole coriander seeds (optional)

INSTRUCTIONS

1. Prep the chard stalks and leaves: Rinse out the Swiss chard leaves thoroughly. Either tear or cut away the thick stalks from the leaves.

2. Cut the stalk pieces into 1-inch pieces. Chop the leaves into inch-wide strips. Keep the stalks and leaves separate.

3. Sauté garlic and crushed red pepper flakes: Heat the olive oil in a sauté pan on medium high heat. Add garlic slices, crushed red pepper, and coriander seeds (if using), and cook for about 30 seconds, or until the garlic is fragrant.

4. Add Swiss chard stalks: Add the chopped Swiss chard stalks. Lower the heat to low, cover and cook for 3 to 4 minutes.

5. Add the chopped leaves: Add the chopped chard leaves, toss with the oil and garlic in the pan. Cover and cook for 3 to 4 more minutes. Turn the leaves and the stalks over in the pan.

6. If the chard still needs a bit more cooking (remove a piece and taste it), cover and cook a few more minutes.

7. Serve immediately.

Buck wheat

Preparation time

15 minutes

INGREDIENTS

- 160 g Buckwheat groats

Instructions

1. Place the buckwheat groats in a medium to large saucepan (with enough room for the buckwheat and lots of water).

2. Pour over plenty of boiling water from the kettle.

3. Bring to the boil over a high heat, then turn down the heat to medium-low and cook for 10-15 minutes, depending on your personal preferences. I recommend testing after 10 minutes and if it's not quite cooked enough for your tastes, cook it a little longer.

4. Drain the buckwheat in a sieve and serve.

5. Notes

6. Many recipes suggest rinsing the buckwheat, either before or after cooking. However, from extensive testing I have discovered this is not necessary so long as you cook the buckwheat in lots of freshly boiled water.

7. Suitable for freezing.

Wheat bran

Preparation time

I hour 45 minutes

INGREDIENTS

- 3 cups bread flour

- 4 or 5 tbsp wheat bran

- 25 g fresh yeast

- 1/2 tsp salt

- 250 ml water

INSTRUCTIONS

1. In a large bowl, mix flour with salt and wheat bran.

2. Dissolve the fresh yeast in water and add to the flour mixture.

3. Mix everything together and knead until the dough is smooth and pulls away from the side of the bowl.

4. Grease a 8 inch diameter souffle dish.

5. Transfer the dough onto ceramic dish, cover it and let it rise for about 1 hour.

6. Preheat the oven to 220°C (430°F) 30 minutes before baking.

7. Put the ceramic dish in the oven and bake for 10 minutes then reduce heat to 190°C (370°F) and bake for another 15-20 minutes.

8. For the last 2,3 minutes use the grill function of the oven to obtain a golden crust.

9. When ready let the bread cool on a rack before serving.

Brazil nut

Preparation time

15 minutes

INGREDIENTS

1 Brazil nut

INSTRUCTIONS

Raw

1. Break off the nut from it's shell

2. Rinse and eat

To cook Brazil nuts on the stovetop:

1. Place a layer of Brazil nuts in a skillet over medium heat.

2. Stir the nuts every minute or so to avoid burning them.

3. Continue cooking for about 5 to 10 minutes until the nuts become aromatic.

To roast Brazil nuts in the oven:

1. Preheat the oven to 350°F.

2. Place the nuts on a layer of parchment paper on a baking sheet.

3. Place the baking sheet in the preheated oven and roast for 5 minutes.

4. Remove the baking sheet and stir the nuts.

5. Return the baking sheet to the oven for another 5 minutes.

6. Remove the nuts from the oven and season them with salt, herbs, or spices.

7. Allow the nuts to cool completely before eating them.

Apricot juice

Preparation time

15 minutes

INGREDIENTS

- 1 kg – 2.2 lbs apricots

- 150 gr – 2/3 cup sugar

- 1 lt – 4 cups water

- 2 lemons

INSTRUCTIONS

1. Carefully wash the apricots.

2. Remove the pits and cut them into small cubes.

3. Put the water and the sugar together in a pot and cook until the syrup reaches a boil.

4. Add the apricots and the lemon and continue cooking for another 10 minutes until they are soft.

5. Blend everything together with an immersion blender until smooth and creamy. At this point, if

you prefer, pour the mixture through a strainer to remove the pulp.

Red grape juice

Preparation time

10 minutes

INGREDIENTS

- 2 LBS grapes

- water

- sugar/ honey

- mesh strainer, to strain unwanted pulp

INSTRUCTIONS

1. Wash grapes and take them off the vines. Make sure they're sparkling clean!

2. Now that the grapes are washed, place your water into the blender and sugar/ honey.

3. Add the grapes.

4. on your smoothie or juicing setting. I usually run 2 cycles of this to make sure there are not clumps at all.

5. There will be bits of skin and pulp remaining in the juice. You can 100% drink the juice like this! Using a fine strainer pour the juice through the strainer to remove the pulp.

Lemon juice

Preparation time

10 minutes

Ingredients

- 1 cup white, granulated sugar (can reduce to 3/4 cup)

- 1 cup water (for the simple syrup)

- 1 cup lemon juice

- 2 to 3 cups cold water (to dilute)

INSTRUCTIONS

1. Make "simple syrup":

2.   Place the sugar and water in a small saucepan and bring to a simmer.

3. Stir so that the sugar dissolves completely and remove from heat.

4. Juice the lemons: While the water is heating for the simple syrup, juice your lemons.

5. Depending on the size of the lemons, 4 to 6 of them should be enough for one cup of juice.

6. Combine lemon juice, simple syrup, water: Pour the juice and the simple syrup sugar water into a serving pitcher.

7. Add 2 to 3 cups of cold water and taste.

8. Add more water if you would like it to be more diluted (though note that when you add

ice, it will melt and naturally dilute the lemonade).

9. If the lemonade is a little sweet for your taste, add a little more straight lemon juice to it.

10. Chill: Refrigerate 30 to 40 minutes.

11. with ice, sliced lemons.

Papaya juice

Preparation time

10 minutes

INGREDIENTS

• 1 ripe medium-size pawpaw

- 1 lemon juiced

- 4 cups water

- Ice cubes for serving

- Sweetener to taste Sugar, Honey, Maple syrup, or any other sweetener of your choice

Instructions

1. Peel the pawpaw and use a spoon to scrape out the seeds from the core. Cut into small chunks.

2. Put the chunks inside a blender.

3. Add the water, lemon juice, and sweetener and blend till smooth.

4. Keep refrigerated, chilled till serving and enjoy with ice cubes.

Banana juice

Preparation time

10 minutes

INGREDIENTS

• large Bananas, sliced

• 1/2 Apple, cored and chopped

• 1 tablespoon Honey

• 1½ cups Milk or Water (milk is preferable)

INSTRUCTIONS

1. Wash the bananas and apple, and pat dry them.

2. Peel the banana and cut into sliced. Peel the apple and cut into halves. Take one portion and cut into smaller pieces, keep the other portion for late use.

3. Add banana chunks, apple pieces and honey into the blender jar.

4. Add milk then blend all ingredients together until smooth puree

5. Add more milk if it's too thick.

6. Then blend for another 5 seconds.

7. Pour into serving glasses, garnish with a banana wheel and serve.

Wild salmon

Preparation time

20 minutes

INGREDIENTS

- 2 (3 ounce) fillets salmon, with skin

- sea salt to taste

- 2 tablespoons olive oil

INSTRUCTIONS

1. Rinse the salmon fillets and pat dry thoroughly with paper towels; season with sea salt.

2. Heat the oil in a skillet over medium-high heat.

3. Gently lay the salmon into the hot oil with the skin side facing up and cook until the the flesh side is golden brown, 5 to 7 minutes; turn and continue cooking until the skin side is slightly browned, about 5 minutes more.

4. Remove the salmon from the skillet, allowing any oil to drain from the fish back into the pan.

5. Remove the skin from the salmon fillets; fry the skin in the oil remaining in the skillet until crispy, 2 to 3 minutes.

6. Serve the crispy skin with the salmon.

Down - Regulation IVF Smoothie

Preparation time

6 minutes

INGREDIENTS

- 2 cups organic baby leaf spinach (lightly steamed)

- 1 organic kiwi fruit

- ½ avocado (freeze the other half for use later)

- 1 tbsp chia seeds

- 1 pinch unrefined sea salt (I prefer Himalayan rose pink salt)

- 1 cup filtered water

- 1 tbsp organic vanilla coconut yogurt (I like COYO)

- 1 tbsp collagen powder

- 1 tsp pure vanilla bean powder

- 1 tsp organic cold pressed avocado oil (optional)

INSTRUCTIONS

1. Prep the spinach first

2. Place the spinach in a colander or steaming basket over a saucepan of barely simmering

water, pop a lid on and steam gently for 1-2 minutes. Set aside to cool.

3. To make the smoothie

4. Add all ingredients to a blender in the order listed. Blend until smooth. If the smoothie is too thick, add 1 tbsp water at a time until you reach your desired consistency.

EQUIPMENT

- Colander or steaming basket

- Small saucepan

- Measuring cup

* Knife

* Peeler

* Measuring spoons

* High speed blender

NOTES

* I suggest prepping the spinach first so that it has time to cool, you don't want a warm smoothie – gross!

* I usually steam it and then remove from the colander with kitchen tongs, place on a plate lined with kitchen roll and pat dry. I then set aside whilst I prep the other ingredients.

Green Baby smoothie

Preparation time

10 minutes

Ingredients

Brazil Nut Milk:

- 1 cup raw brazil nuts

- 3 cups filtered water

- 2-4 dates, pitted and chopped

- 1 tsp vanilla or 1 vanilla bean pod, chopped

- sprinkle of sea salt

Smoothie:

- 1 - 1 ½ cups Brazil Nut Milk (if not making sub for unsweetened hemp, cashew, almond or coconut milk)

- 1 large handful frozen spinach

- 1 large handful frozen kale

- 1 scoop Vanilla Bone Broth Protein Powder

- 1 tbsp cashew, almond or coconut butter

- 1 tbsp chia seeds

- 1-2 dates, pitted and chopped (depends on how sweet you like it, I prefer two :))

- 1 tsp spirulina powder

- ¼ avocado, pitted, peeled and chopped

- ½ frozen banana

Instructions

1. If making the Brazil Nut Milk (delicious and supports optimal thyroid function) soak ALL nut milk ingredients in a bowl overnight, or for at least 8 hours. When done soaking, mix well in a high speed blender, then pour through a fine mesh strainer or nut milk bag (you will want to do this to remove small particles, otherwise the texture of the milk won't be as smooth).

2. If making the Brazil nut milk, use as a base of the smoothie (if not sub an alternative unsweetened nut milk) and add in all other ingredients to a high speed blender and mix until smooth.

3. This recipe makes a really thick, creamy smoothie (just the way I like it) but if you like smoothies on the more liquid-side, try adding more milk to thin the consistency.

4. Top with desired toppings. I love adding a dollop of probiotic-rich coconut yogurt, sprinkle of paleo granola and scoop of cashew butter.

Berrylicious Fruit Crumble

Ingredients

For the Fruit Filling:

- 2 1/2 cups strawberries chopped (fresh or frozen, about 16 ounces)

- 1 cup raspberries fresh or frozen, 6 ounces

- 1 tablespoon granulated sugar

- 11/2 teaspoons lemon juice

- 1/2 teaspoon lemon zest

- 2 tablespoons white whole wheat flour

For the Oat Crumble Topping:

- 2 tablespoons white whole wheat flour

- 2/3 cup rolled old fashioned oats

- 1 tablespoon brown sugar packed

- 3/4 teaspoon ground cinnamon

- 1/4 teaspoon kosher salt

- 1 tablespoon melted butter or 1 tablespoon vegetable oil

- 1 tablespoon whole milk

- 1 1/2 teaspoon vanilla extract

- 2 tablespoons chopped walnuts

Instructions

1. Preheat oven to 375°F

2. In a medium bowl, mix together strawberries, raspberries, sugar, lemon juice and lemon zest.

3. Place fruit mixture into a 9-inch pie pan sprayed with nonstick spray.

4. Cover with foil and bake for 20 minutes.

5. While baking, mix flour, oats, brown sugar, cinnamon and salt in a bowl, and set aside.

6. In a small bowl, whisk together the butter (or vegetable oil), milk and vanilla.

7. Pour the wet ingredients into the dry and blend together using the back of a fork as a pastry blender, mixing until dry ingredients are well coated.

8. Mix in the chopped walnuts and sprinkle the remaining oat crumble topping over the top of the pie dish.

9. Continue to bake, uncovered, for remaining 15 to 20 minutes, until fruit bubbles at the top. Remove and let cool for 10 to 15 minutes before serving.

10. Variation: Substitute 1½ pounds pitted sweet cherries, cut in half, ½ teaspoon almond extract for vanilla extract, and sliced almonds for the walnuts.

Storage:

Refrigerate in a sealed container for up to 3 days.

Herbal Fertility Tea

Preparation time

20 minutes

Ingredients

- 2 cups red raspberry leaf

- 1 cup dried stinging nettle leaf

- 1 cup dried peppermint

- 1 cup red clover

- 1/2 cup green tea leaves optional

Instructions

1. Combine all herbs and optional green tea into a bowl.

2. Stir to combine and store in an airtight container away from direct sunlight.

To drink as a tea:

1. Add 1/4 cup herb blend to a coffee or tea press.

2. Add boiling water, cover, and allow to steep for 10 minutes.

3. Discard used herbs, then enjoy tea in a mug with a touch of honey or a lemon slice.

To drink as an infusion:

1. Add 1/2 cup herb blend to a quart-sized Mason jar.

2. Fill with tepid water to top. Close the jar and leave at room temperature overnight.

3. In the morning, pour infusion through a strainer into another quart-sized Mason jar.

4. Discard herbs and drink infusion as desired!

5. Store in the refrigerator if it will not be consumed within 12 hours.

Berry Smoothie

Preparation time

10 minutes

Ingredients:

* 1 banana

* 3 spoonfuls of kefir yoghurt

* 3 spoonfuls of oats

* Handful of almonds

* Spoonful of linseeds

* Berries (like blueberries, raspberries, strawberries)

- Milk (or dairy free alternative like almond milk)

Instructions

1. One easy step – blend all together and enjoy!

Winter Warmer Squash Soup

Preparation time

60 minutes

Ingredients:

- 2 tbsp olive oil

- sprig of rosemary (or can used dried)

- 3 garlic cloves

- 1/2 medium chilli, finely chopped

- 1 medium butternut squash, peeled and cubed

- 2 carrots, peeled and cubed

- 1 large potato, chopped

- 2 celery sticks, peeled and cubed

- 1 medium onion, chopped

- pinch cumin seeds

- 1/2 tsp chilli flakes

- pinch smoked paprika

- 2 pints veg stock

Instructions

1. Heat oil in a large saucepan

2. Add garlic, chilli, paprika, rosemary and cumin seeds and heat for 30 seconds (do not colour, you only want to release the flavours).

3. Add all the vegetables – you do not need to worry about chopping them too finely, as you are going to blend them

4. Soften the vegetables for 2 minutes until they are fully coated in the spices.

5. Add the stock, turn down the heat and allow the soup to simmer for about 45 mins.

6. Once cooked blend with a hand whisk.

7. Season to taste (if you like spice, you might want to add more chilli!)

8. To serve – sprinkle with feta and pumpkin seeds.

Salmon Couscous Parcel

Preparation time

40 minutes

Ingredients:

- 110g of couscous

- 200ml hot vegetable stock

- 1 tbsp olive oil

- Handful of chopped herbs (parsley, dill, rosemary – or whatever you have in fridge)

- Grilled vegetables (courgette/ pepper)

- 4 Sundried tomatoes

- 2 salmon fillets, approx 140g/5oz each

Instructions

1. Preheat oven to 200C/fan 180C/gas 6.

2. Put the couscous in a bowl and stir in the oil and stock.

3. Cover and leave to stand 10 minutes until the stock is absorbed.

4. While the couscous is standing, cook the vegetables – either in the grill or on a griddle pan.

5. In terms of quantities one courgette or pepper is plenty.

6. Fluff the cous cous with a fork, and then add in the chopped herbs, sundried tomatoes and grilled vegetables.

7. Divide the couscous between two sheets of baking paper.

8. Sit the salmon fillets on the couscous, and season with salt and pepper (you can add some slices of lemon on top if you like).

9. Fold the paper over, then twist the edges together creating a little parcel.

10. Put the parcels onto a baking tray and bake for 15 mins or until the fish feels firm to the touch.

Lemon Ginger Smoothie

Preparation time

10 minutes

INGREDIENTS

- 1 whole organic lemon

- 1 large knob of fresh ginger, peeled (I do about the size of my thumb, but you could do less)

- 1 tbsp organic walnut oil (or other fat- coconut butter, fish oil, flax oil)

- 2 tsp organic sunflower lecithin (NOT SOY LECITHIN!!!!)

- 1 capsule Vitamin E 100 IU Mixed Tocopherols

- 1 ¾ cup filtered water

- Optional: Add 1/2 tsp of organic ceylon cinnamon (especially good for those with PCOS)

INSTRUCTIONS

1. Gently scrub the lemon to make sure it is clean- we use this natural scrubber with coconut bristles and love it.

2. Put all the ingredients into your Nutribullet tall cup or other blender.

3. Blend for 30 seconds.

4. Strain through a fine mesh strainer (we use one from this set).

5. I use a spoon to help push it through, because I lack patience.

6. Pour into two glass containers- one to drink now, and one that you can put a top on (like a pint size mason jar) and put in the fridge for later.

7. Drink the second within 24 hours!

Citrus and Banana Smoothie

Preparation time

30 minutes

Ingredients

- 2 Ripe banana, peeled and sliced

- 1/2 cup water

- 2 oranges, peeled and sliced

- 3 cups plain Greek yogurt use nut-based yogurt if you are vegan

- 2 tbsp grated orange zest (from orange)

- 2 tsp pure vanilla extract

- 1 cup ice

- 1/2 cup sugar optional

Instructions

1. Make sure you have a strong, powerful blender that will blend all the ingredients. I like using Ninja Master Prep Professional!

2. In a small saucepan, bring the sugar and water to a boil over medium-high heat. Simmer and stir occasionally until the sugar dissolves, which would be about 5 minutes.

3. Cool for 20 minutes.

4. Add the Greek yogurt, banana,oranges, orange zest, vanilla extract, and ice.

5. Blend until the mixture is thick, creamy and smooth (around 3 minutes)

6. Pour into glasses and serve.

Indonesian Chicken with Buckwheat Noodles

Preparation time

90 minutes

Ingredients

- 1 lemongrass stalk, chopped

- 1 handful of coriander leaves

- 1 small onion, chopped

- 2 garlic cloves, crushed

- 2cm/¾in piece root ginger, peeled and grated

- 1 tbsp coconut sugar or honey

- 1 tbsp soy sauce

- 1 tbsp fish sauce

- ½ tsp turmeric

- 1 tsp garam masala

- 400ml/14fl oz/generous 1½ cups coconut milk

- 4 skinless boneless chicken thighs, cut into large chunks

- 125g/4½oz buckwheat noodles

- 1 tsp sesame oil

- 1 tbsp coconut oil

- 1 red chilli, deseeded and diced

- 1 pak choi, cut into strips

- 100g/3½oz mangetout

- 4 shiitake mushrooms, sliced

- sea salt and ground black pepper

- 1 handful of bean sprouts, to serve

- 2 spring onions, chopped, to serve

Instructions

1. Put the lemongrass, coriander, onion, garlic, ginger, coconut sugar, soy sauce, fish sauce, turmeric, garam masala and coconut milk in a blender or food processor and process until smooth.

2. Pour over the chicken pieces and season lightly with salt and pepper.

3. Cover and leave to marinate in the fridge for at least 2 hours, or overnight.

4. Cook the buckwheat noodles with the sesame oil according to the packet instructions, then drain and refresh under cold water.

5. Meanwhile, heat the coconut oil in a wok or large frying pan.

6. Drain the chicken, reserving the marinade, and stir-fry for 2–3 minutes.

7. Add the chilli, pak choi, mangetout and mushrooms and cook for a further 1 minute.

8. Add the reserved marinade and simmer for 10–15 minutes until the chicken is cooked through.

9. Toss in the noodles and warm through.

10. Sprinkle over the bean sprouts and spring onions and serve.

Egg and Spinach Salad

Preparation time

20 minutes

Ingredients

- 4 large British Lion eggs

- 60ml/4tbsp vegetable oil

- 50g/2oz ciabatta or other crusty bread

- 2 ripe tomatoes, roughly chopped

- 50g/2oz sunblush tomatoes in oil plus 30ml/2tbsp of the oil from the tomatoes

- 6 basil leaves, shredded

- 100g/4oz baby spinach leaves

Instructions

1. Place 3 eggs in a small pan, cover with boiling water and bring to the boil.

2. Boil for 6 mins, drain the eggs, rinse in cold water, tapping the shells all over.

3. When cool enough to handle, peel away the shells. Cut into quarters.

4. Heat the oil in a frying pan until hot.

5. Tear the ciabatta into bite sized pieces and add to the hot oil.

6. Fry for 2 to 3 mins, stirring occasionally until the croutons are crisp and golden.

7. Drain on kitchen paper.

8. Mix the tomatoes together with the oil and basil.

9. Season to taste.

10. Empty the spinach into 2 serving bowls, add the croutons, quartered eggs and tomatoes.

11. Toss together and serve

Shakshuka(Egg in tomatoes sauce)

Preparation time

Ingredients:

- 1 tablespoon olive oil

* ½ cup (2 ounces) onion, chopped

* 1 medium (5 ounces) bell pepper (any color), chopped

* 2 cloves garlic, minced

* ½ teaspoon black pepper

* ¾ teaspoon Italian seasoning

* 1/8 teaspoon kosher salt

* 1 can (28 ounces) diced tomatoes, no salt added

* 4 large eggs

* Red pepper flakes (optional garnish)

Instructions:

1. Place a large nonstick skillet over medium heat.

2. Add olive oil, onion, and bell peppers.

3. Cook 5 to 7 minutes, or until softened.

4. Add the minced garlic, black pepper, Italian seasoning, and kosher salt. Stir and cook for 2 to 3 minutes, then add the tomatoes.

5. Turn heat to medium, cover, and let cook for 5 minutes.

6. Remove lid and create four small holes in the tomato mixture.

7. Crack an egg into each hole, then cover and cook for an additional 6 minutes, until white is firm and yolk is set but still able to be punctured

with a fork. (If you prefer a set egg with a firm yolk, cook for 8 minutes.)

8. Remove from heat and serve.

Quinoa with Cumin and Lime

Preparation time

30 minutes

INGREDIENTS

- 1 tablespoon olive oil

- 1 cup quinoa, rinsed thoroughly

- 1 tablespoon ground cumin

- 2 cups water

- 1 lime, juice and zest

- ¼ cup chopped fresh cilantro

- Salt and freshly ground black pepper, to taste

INSTRUCTIONS

1. Set a medium saucepan over medium-high heat and add the olive oil.

2. Once the oil is hot, add the quinoa and toast for 1-2 minutes, stirring constantly.

3. Add cumin and continue to stir, cooking an additional minute.

4. Add the water and bring to a boil.

5. Reduce the heat and simmer, stirring occasionally, until quinoa is cooked, about 15-20 minutes.

6. Drain any excess water.

7. Add the lime juice and zest, cilantro, salt and pepper and toss until well combined.

Baked Mediterranean Chicken Recipe

Preparation time

45 minutes

Ingredients

- 1 can (12 ounces) no salt added diced tomatoes, liquids and solids

- 2 cloves garlic, chopped

- 1 tsp dried oregano

- ⅓ rounded cup Kalamata olives, chopped (about 16 olives)

- 4 boneless, skinless chicken breasts (1 ¼ pound)

- ¼ cup crumbled feta cheese

Instructions

1. Preheat the oven to 400°F.

2. Combine diced tomatoes, garlic, oregano, and olives in a mixing bowl and set aside.

3. Coat a 9x13-inch glass baking dish with nonstick cooking spray.

4. Place chicken breasts evenly in the bottom of the baking dish.

5. Spoon the tomato mixture evenly over the chicken breasts, then sprinkle with feta cheese.

6. Bake in preheated oven for 30 to 35 minutes, or until chicken is cooked through and internal temperature reaches 165°F.

7. Serve immediately

RED AND GREEN FRITTATA

Preparation time

Ingredients

- 6 cups (1.4 liters) bite-size broccoli florets

- 8 large eggs

- 1/4 cup (59 ml) milk

- 1/4 teaspoon (1 ml) salt

- 1/4 teaspoon (1 ml) freshly ground pepper

- 1 red bell pepper, cut into 1/4-inch (6 mm) thick slices

- 1 cup (4 ounces or 113 grams) grated white cheddar or fontina cheese, divided

- 4 tablespoons (60 ml) grated Parmesan cheese, divided

- 2 teaspoons (10 ml) olive oil

Instructions

1. Bring a large pot of water to a boil; add the broccoli and cook until just tender, about 3 minutes. Drain well.

2. Preheat the oven to 350°F (177°C). In a large bowl, whisk the eggs, milk, salt, and pepper together in a large bowl.

3. Stir in the broccoli, red pepper, 3/4 -cup (36 ounces) of the cheddar, and 3 tablespoons (45 ml) of the Parmesan cheese.

4. Heat the oil in a 12-inch (305 mm) ovenproof nonstick frying pan over medium-high heat.

5. Pour the egg mixture into the pan and reduce the heat to medium.

6. Cook for 3 minutes to set the bottom of the frittata.

7. Sprinkle the top with the remaining 1/4 -cup of the Cheddar (12 ounces) and 1 tablespoon (15 ml) Parmesan cheese.

8. Transfer the pan to the oven and bake until the frittata is set in the center and slightly puffed up, about 15 minutes.

9. Let cool for 5 minutes in the pan, and then loosen the edge with a spatula and slide onto a large plate.

10. Cut into wedges and serve warm or at room temperature.

LUNCH: OPEN FACED VEGGIE MELT

(Serves 1)

What You'll Need:

1 slice of hearty, whole-grain bread

Dijon mustard

1 to 2 thin slices red onion

4 to 6 thin slices cucumber

1/2 ripe avocado

Sea salt

Freshly ground pepper

1 slice (about 1 ounce or 28 grams) Swiss cheese

How You'll Make It:

1. Preheat the broiler.

2. Spread the bread generously with mustard. Scoop the avocado flesh from the peel with a spoon and slice lengthwise. Fan the avocado on the mustard. Arrange the onion slices and cucumber over the avocado and sprinkle lightly with salt and pepper. Top with the cheese.

3. Place under the broiler until the cheese is just melted and bubbling, about 1 minute.

CITRUS SHRIMP WITH SUGAR SNAP PEAS

Ingredients

- 2 tablespoons (30 ml) soy sauce

- 1 tablespoon (15 ml) minced peeled fresh ginger

- 1 teaspoon (5 ml) minced orange zest

- 1 clove garlic, minced

- 1/4 teaspoon (1 ml) crushed red pepper flakes

- 1 pound (454 grams) uncooked large shrimp, peeled and deveined

- 11/2 tablespoons (22.5 ml) canola oil

- 4 green onions, cut into thin slices

- 1 pound (454 grams) sugar snap peas, ends trimmed and strings removed

- 1/4 cup (59 ml) chicken broth

- 2 tablespoons (30 ml) fresh orange juice

Instructions

1. In a bowl large enough to hold the shrimp, mix the soy sauce, ginger, orange zest, garlic, and red pepper flakes.

2. Add the shrimp and mix to coat.

3. Chill for 15 minutes.

4. In a large frying pan, heat the oil over high heat.

5. Add the shrimp mixture, green onions, and snap peas.

6. Stir until the shrimp are evenly pink and just opaque in the center, about 2 minutes.

7. Add the broth and orange juice and cook to reduce the sauce slightly, about 1 minute longer.

PARMESAN CHEESE POPCORN

Ingredients

- 3 tablespoons (45 ml) finely shredded Parmesan cheese
- 1 teaspoon (5 ml) smoked paprika

- 1/4 teaspoon (1 ml) ground cumin

- 1/4 teaspoon (1 ml) sea salt

- 6 cups (1.4 liters) popped plain popcorn

- 1/4 cup (59 ml) pumpkin seeds, toasted

- 11/2 tablespoons butter

- Salt and pepper

Instructions

1. In a small bowl, combine the cheese, paprika, cumin, and sea salt.

2. In a large bowl, drizzle the popcorn and pumpkin seeds with the butter and toss well with the Parmesan cheese mixture.

3. Add salt and pepper to taste.

4. Serve immediately.

Tuna Fish

Preparation time

20 minutes

Ingredients

2 pounds albacore tuna (high-quality)

Salt (to taste)

Instructions

With the help of a sharp knife, cut the fish into large chunks about 1-inch thick.

Generously sprinkle the pieces of fish with salt on both sides.

Oatmeal

Preparation time

7 minutes

INGREDIENTS

- 1/2 cup old fashioned oats

- 1 cup milk

- 1/4 teaspoon salt

- 1 tablespoon unsalted butter

Instructions

1. Mix together the oats, milk, salt, and butter into a small saucepan and cook on medium heat.

2. Stir the mixture until it begins to bubble and the oats soften.

3. This should take about 5 minutes and the mixture should look thick and creamy.

4. Add more milk or water if you prefer a thinner oatmeal.

5. Add in any mix-ins that you desire.

6. Sugar, cocoa powder, peanut butter, and mashed peanut butter make great sweet mix-ins to add now.

7. Alternatively, you can consider, cheese and herbs for savory oatmeal.

8. Pour the cooked oats into a bowl.

9. Add in any other mix-ins as desired such as nuts, dried berries, or bacon.

www.ingramcontent.com/pod-product-compliance
Lightning Source LLC
Chambersburg PA
CBHW072102150726
47999CB00005B/1847